Yay! I'm Going Sledding

By Sandy Stream

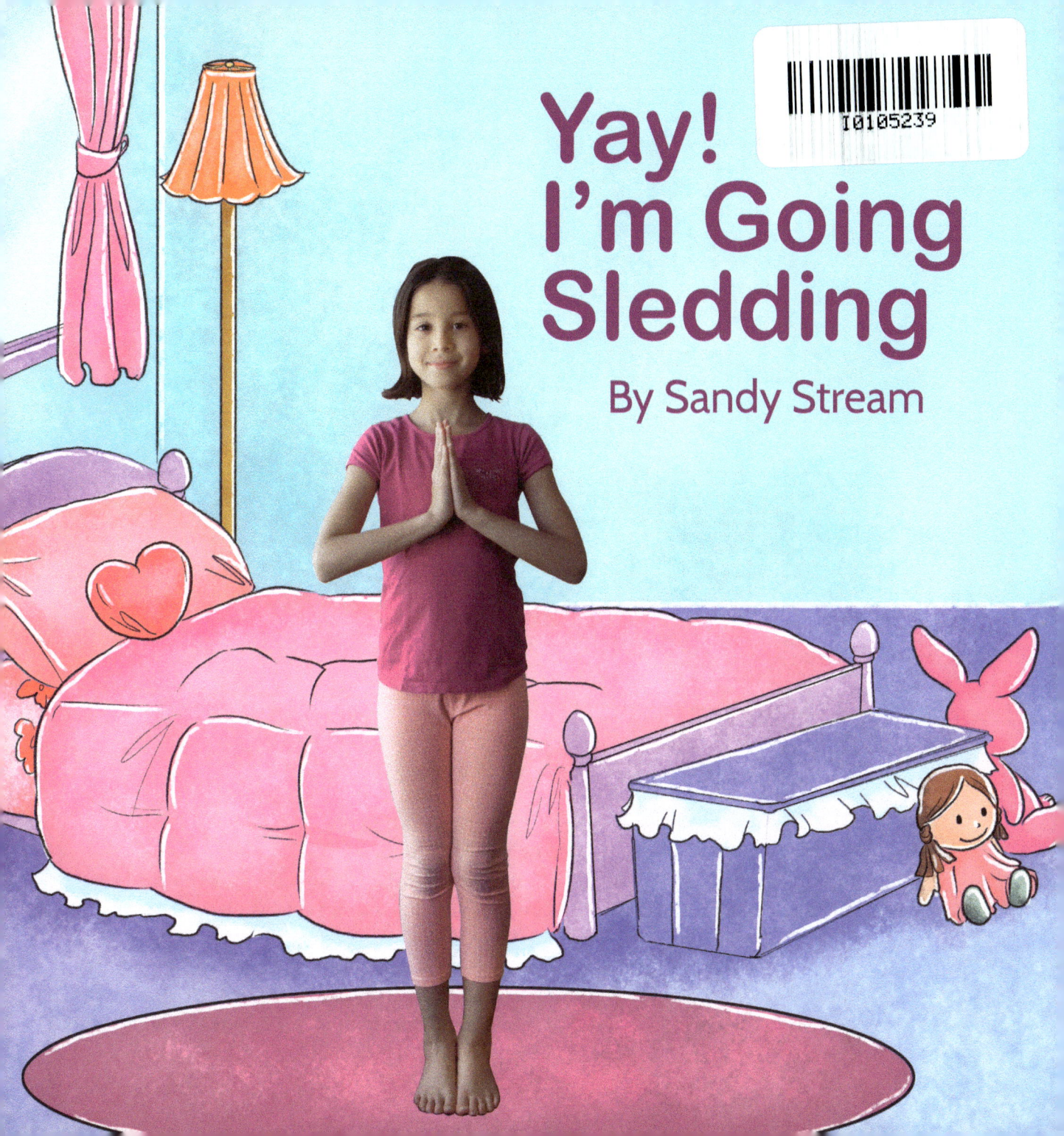

Yay! I'm Going Sledding. By Sandy Stream
Illustrated by Yoko Matsuoka
Edited by Tomoko Matsuoka
Photos: Amelia Bautista. Directed by Juliana Bautista and Paula Kerllenevich
ISBN: 978-0-9938828-1-4

Note to Caregivers

This series is intended to be read to children while encouraging them to try the poses and to be aware of their internal movements and sensations.

Please allow them to do the moves "imperfectly" and to experience the movements in whatever way feels best to them.

To accept ourselves—and to accept what we are feeling inside, whatever it may be—is one of the most fundamental elements on the path towards inner peace.

Hopefully this book serves as one footstep on that path.

Sandy Stream

Once upon a time, there was a little girl named Eve. She woke up so happy because she knew she was going sledding at the park.

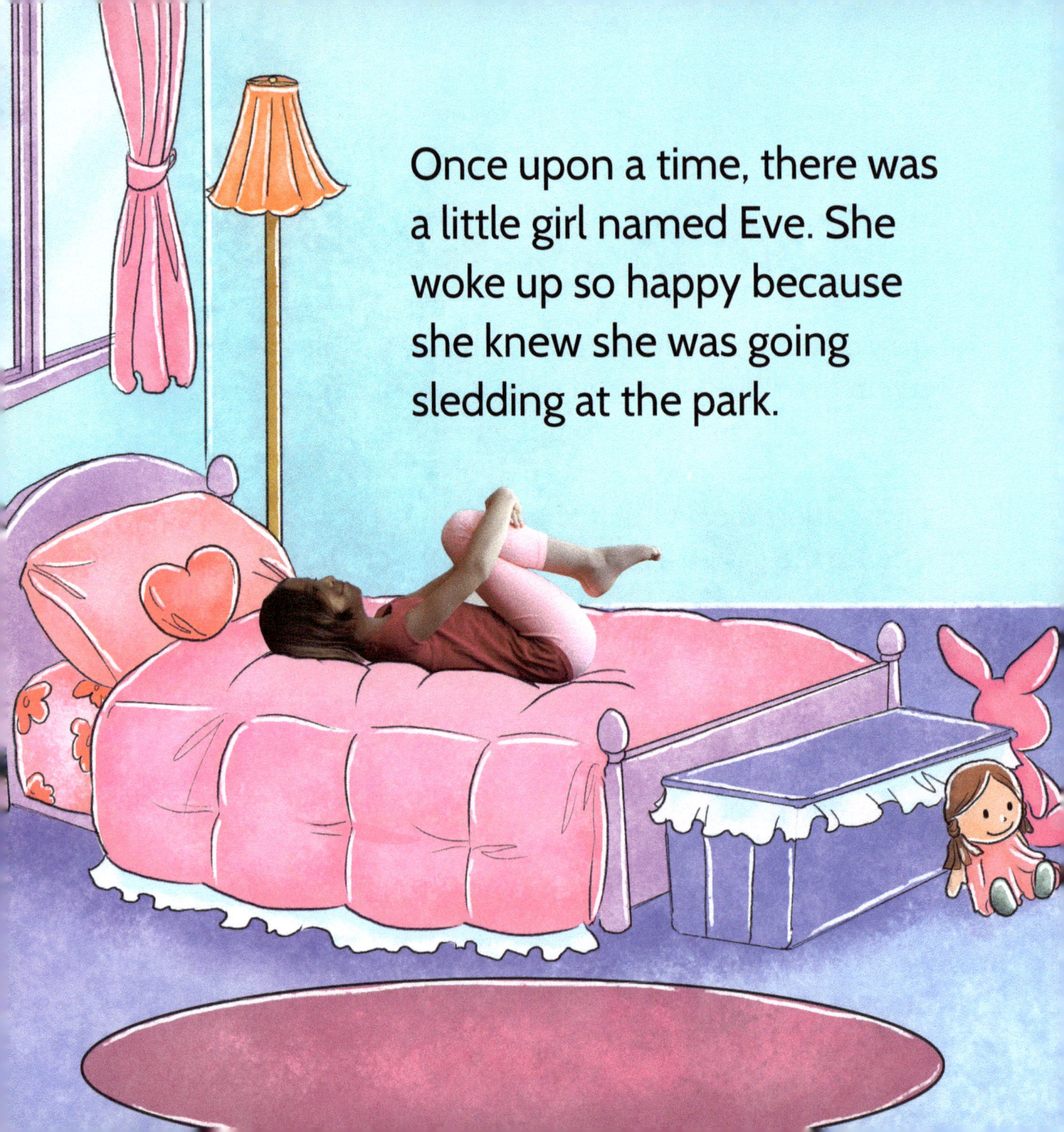

She got up and said good morning to the sun, as she did every morning, and breathed in the fresh air.

Eve loved to play and to explore. She smiled and started getting dressed.

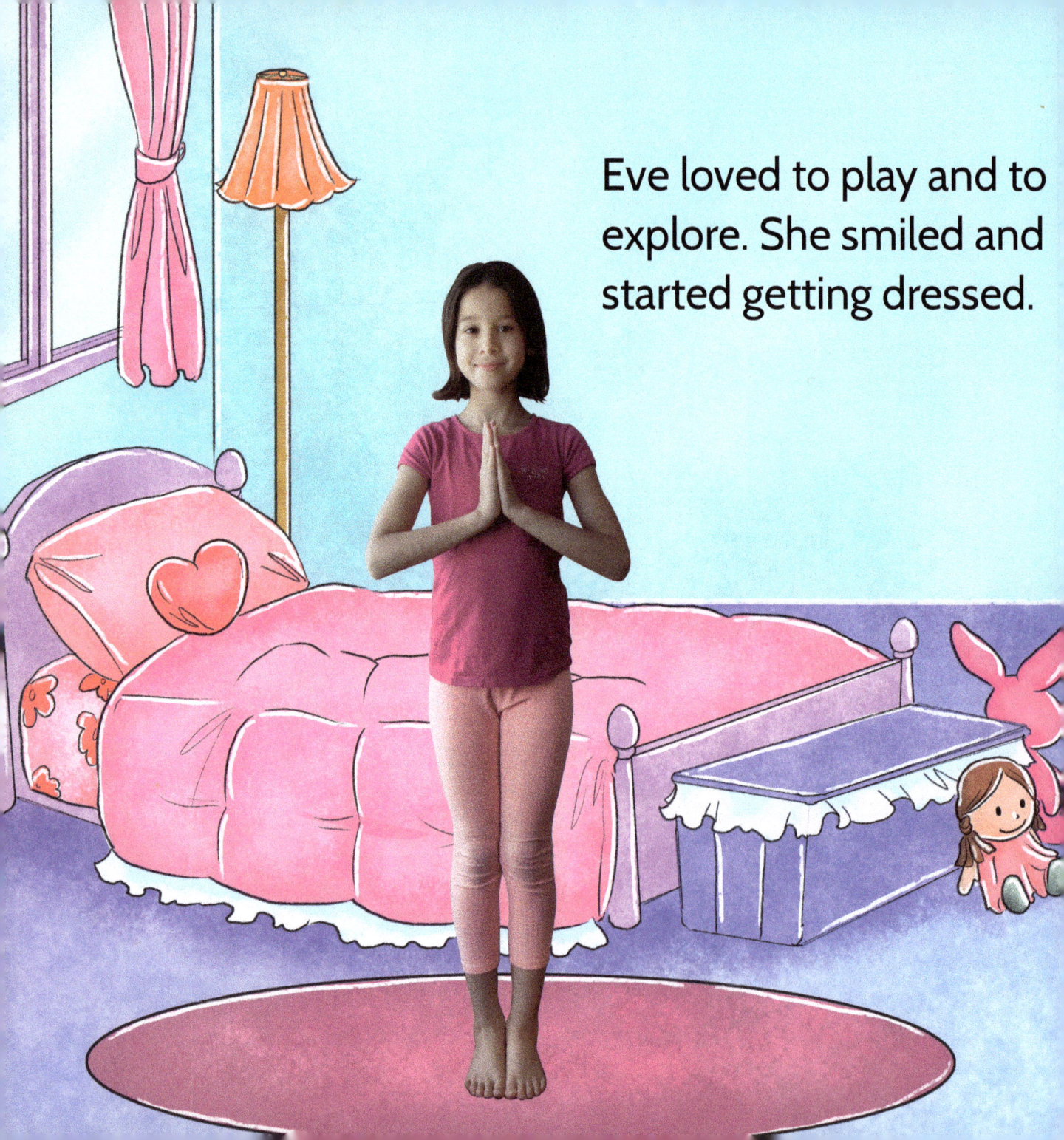

She bent down to
put on one boot,
and then the other.

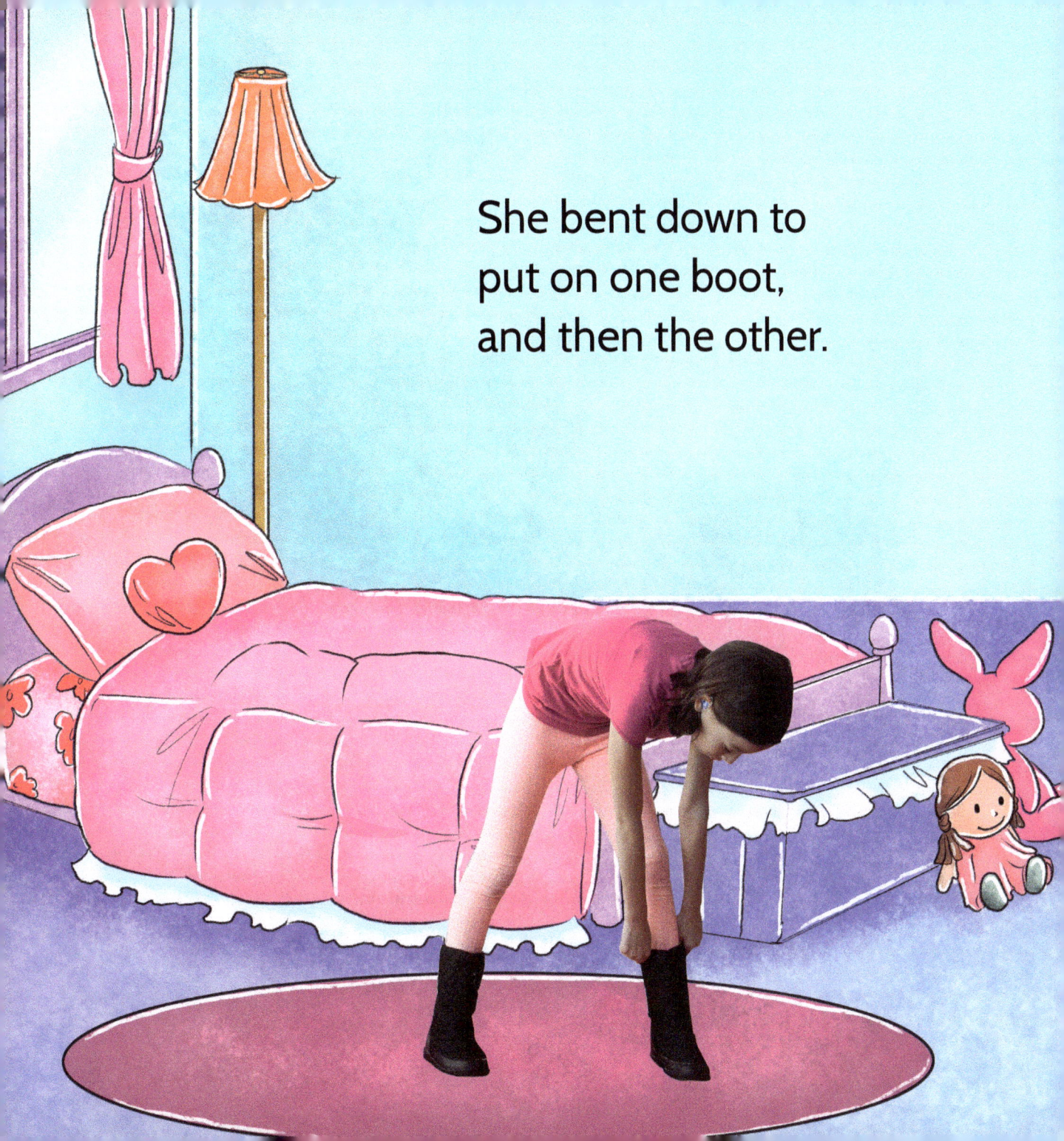

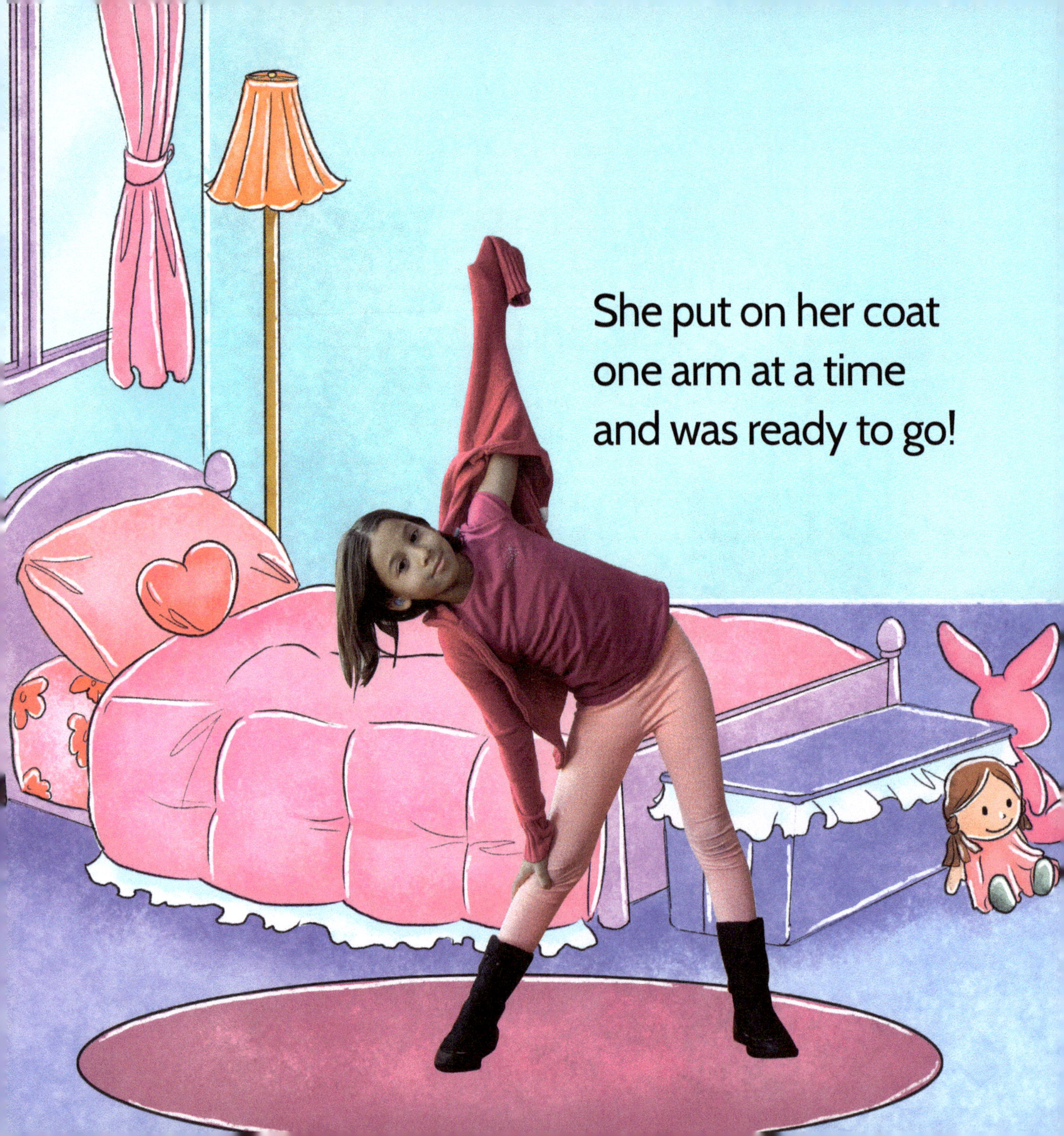

She put on her coat
one arm at a time
and was ready to go!

Off she went to the park.
She looked at the mountain.

Yay! I'm going sledding!

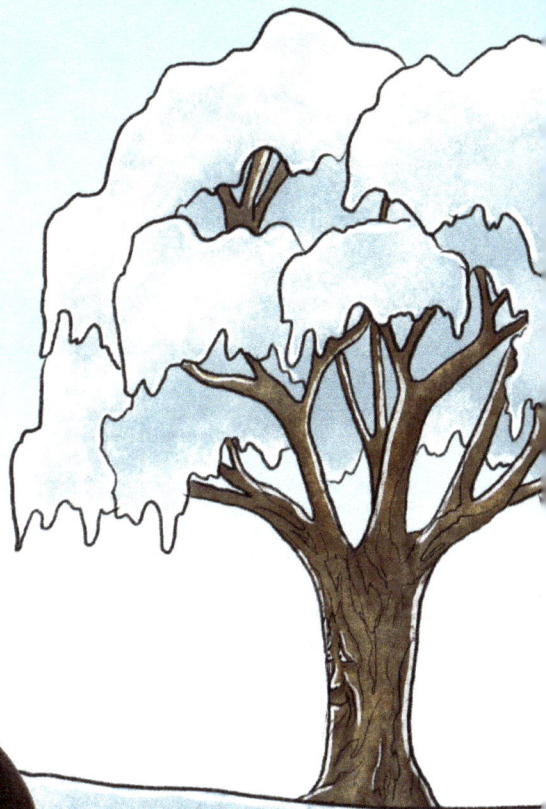

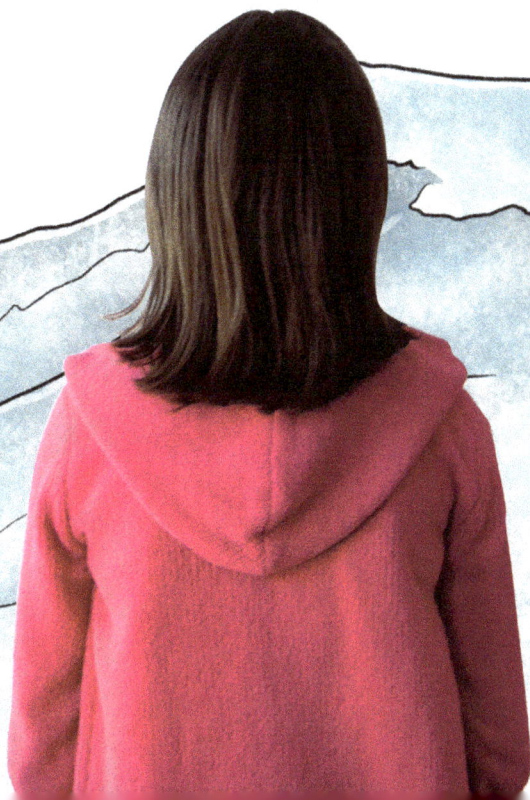

Eve was so excited!

She breathed happily and deeply as she went up the mountain.

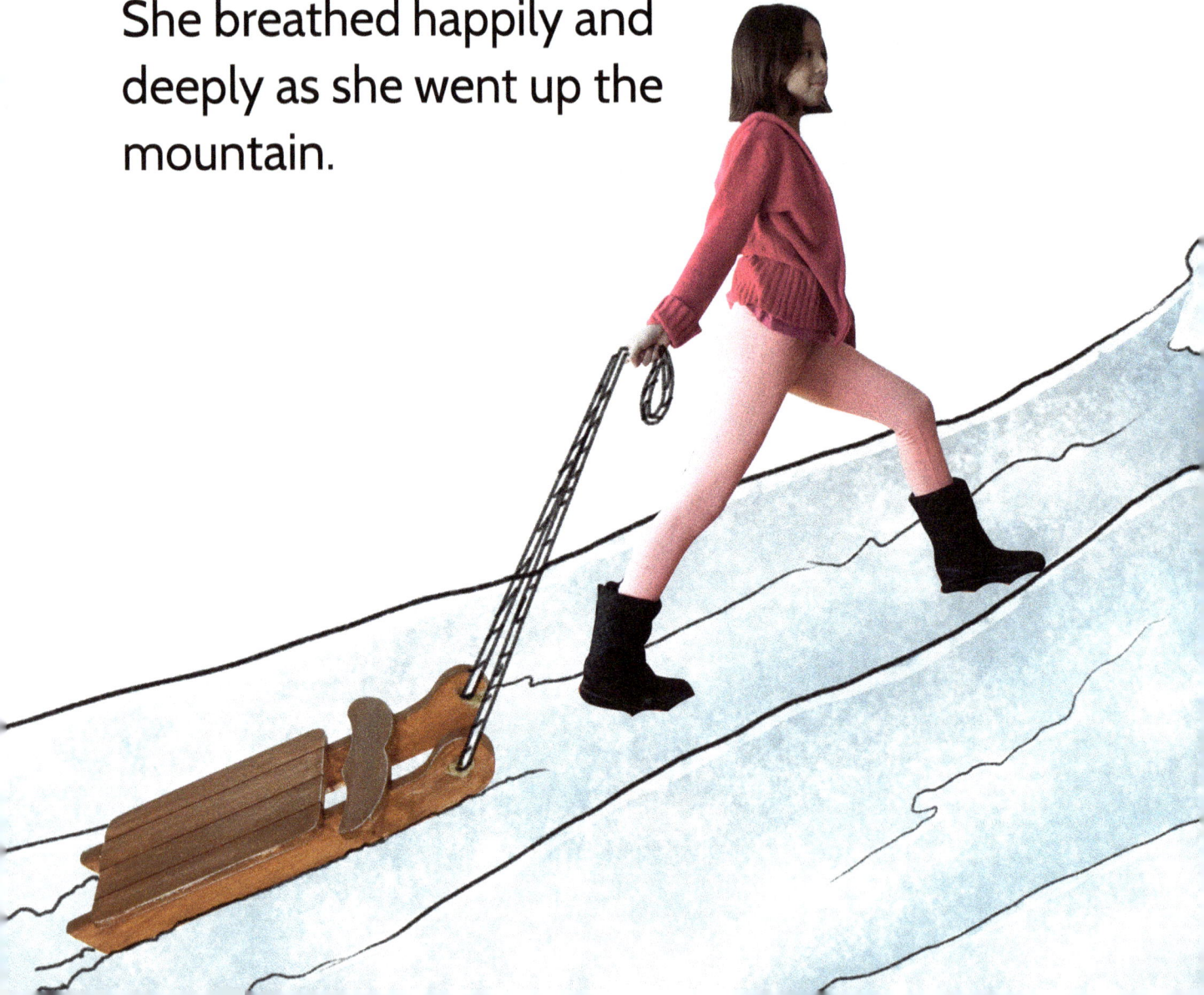

When she reached the top, she was so excited that her heart was beating so fast!

Ba-boom!
Ba-boom!

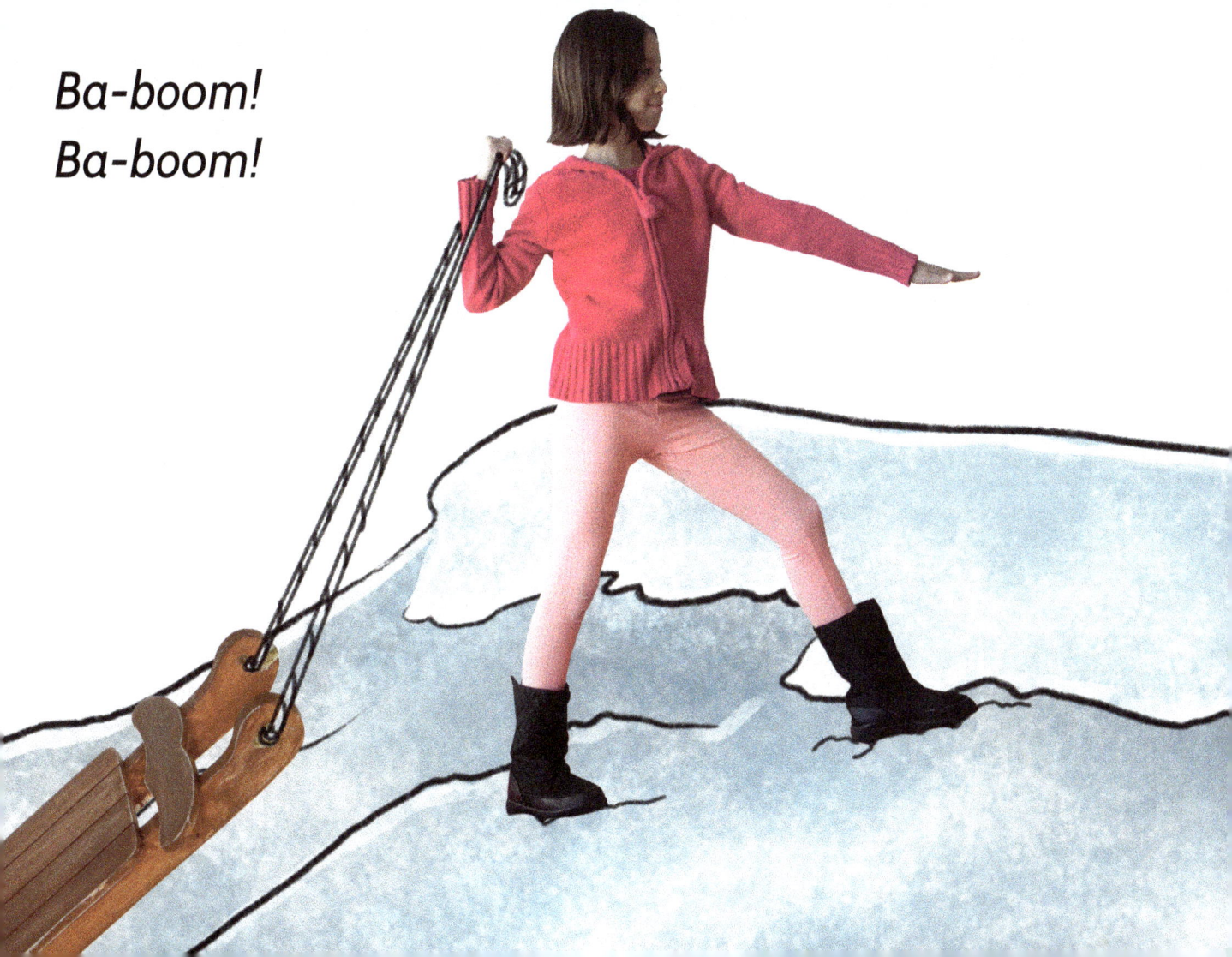

She sat on her sled.
She looked to the left
and to the right to see if
there were any other kids
around.
There were no kids.

That's okay, Eve thought.
She was happy anyway.

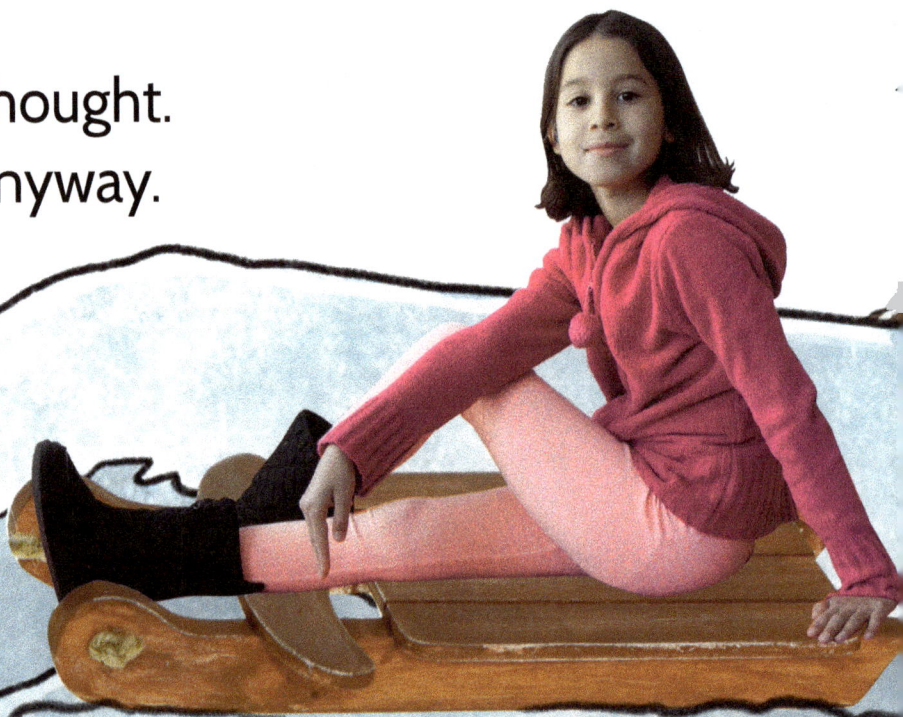

Ready...

Wheeeee!

Her heart was beating so fast,
and she was so happy!

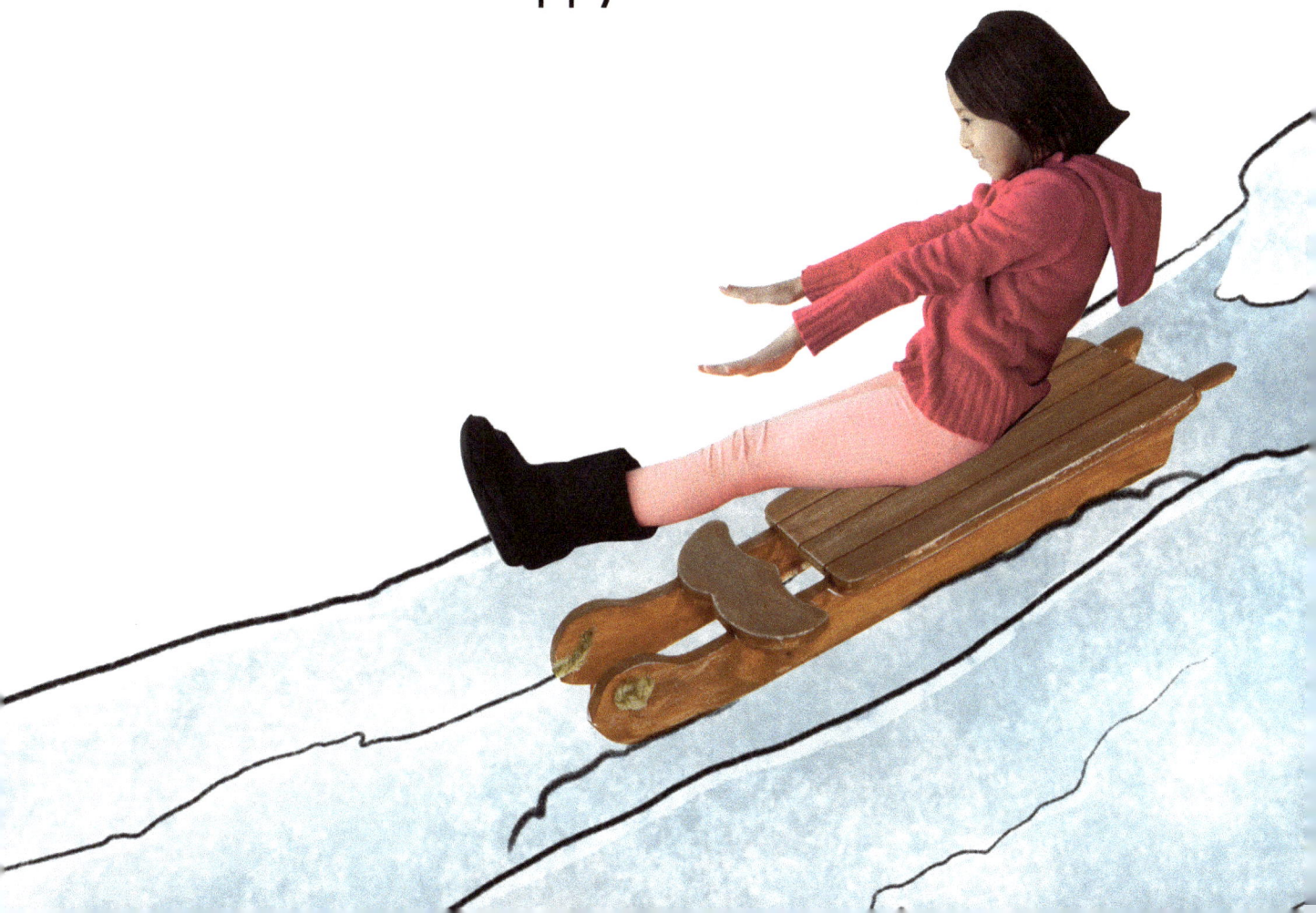

She wanted to go again!

So she climbed
up, up, up,
to the top of the mountain.

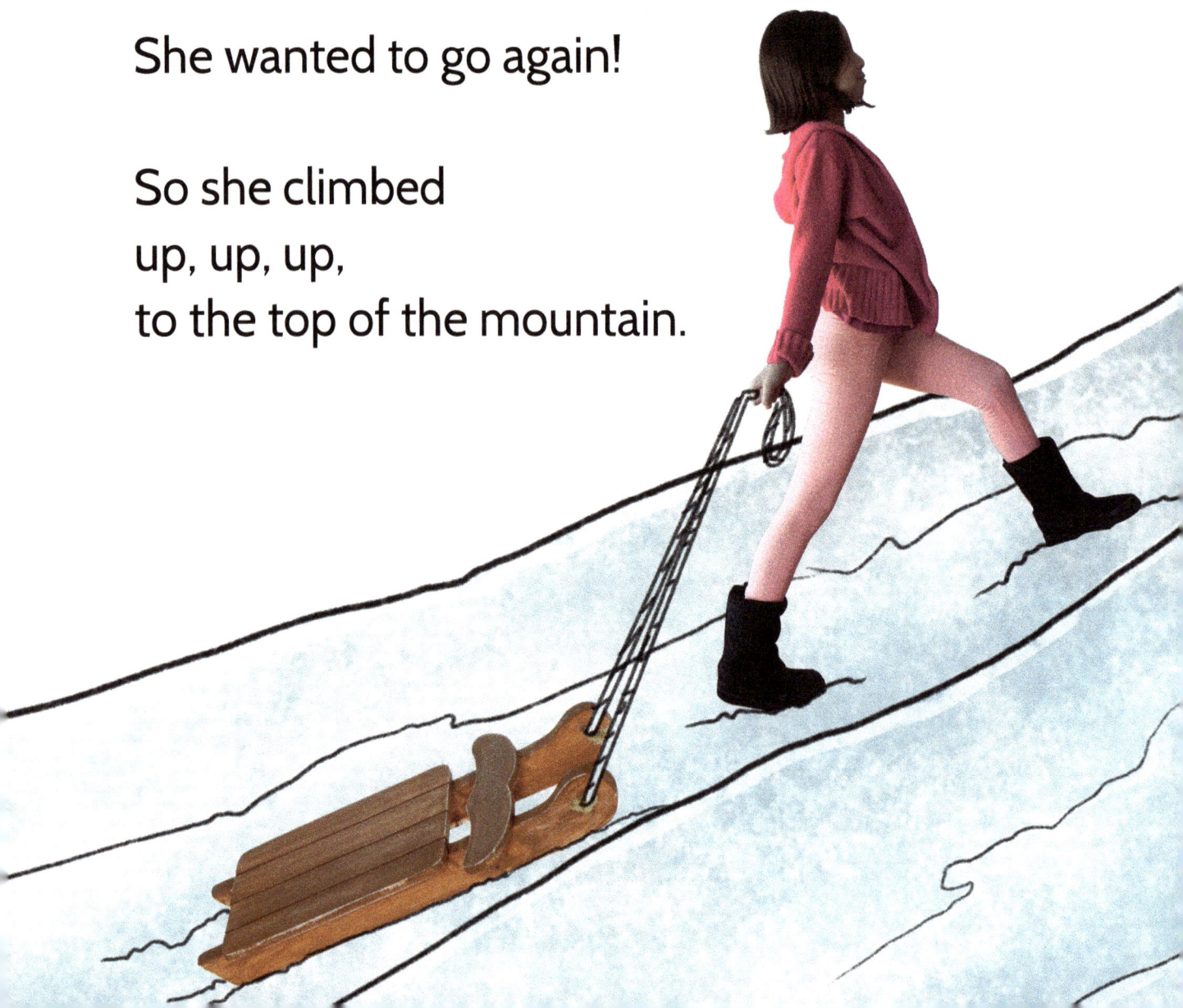

This time she decided to go on her belly.

Wheeeee!

It was so much fun!

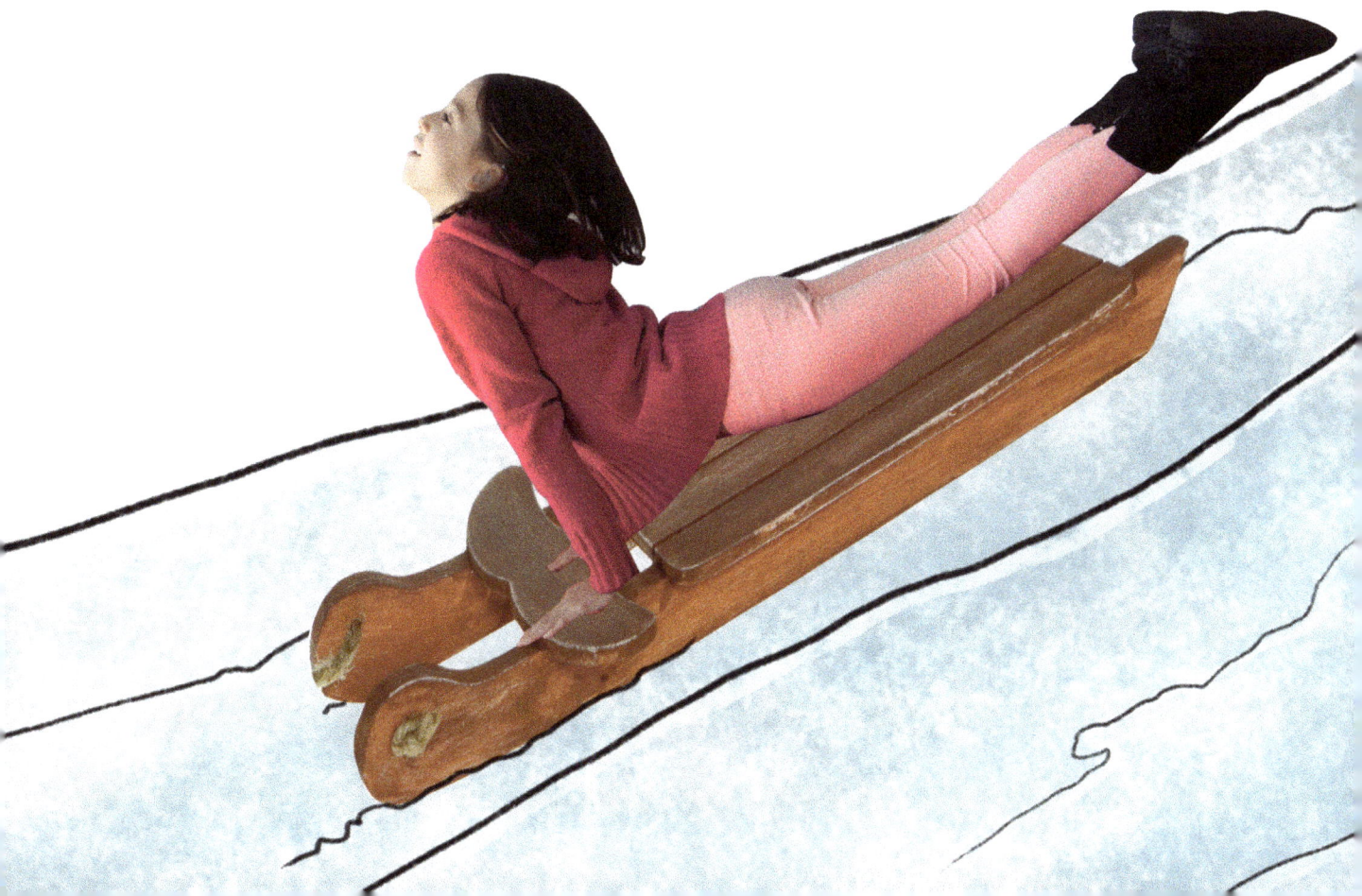

The next time she
climbed up it was a bit
harder because the wind
had begun to blow.

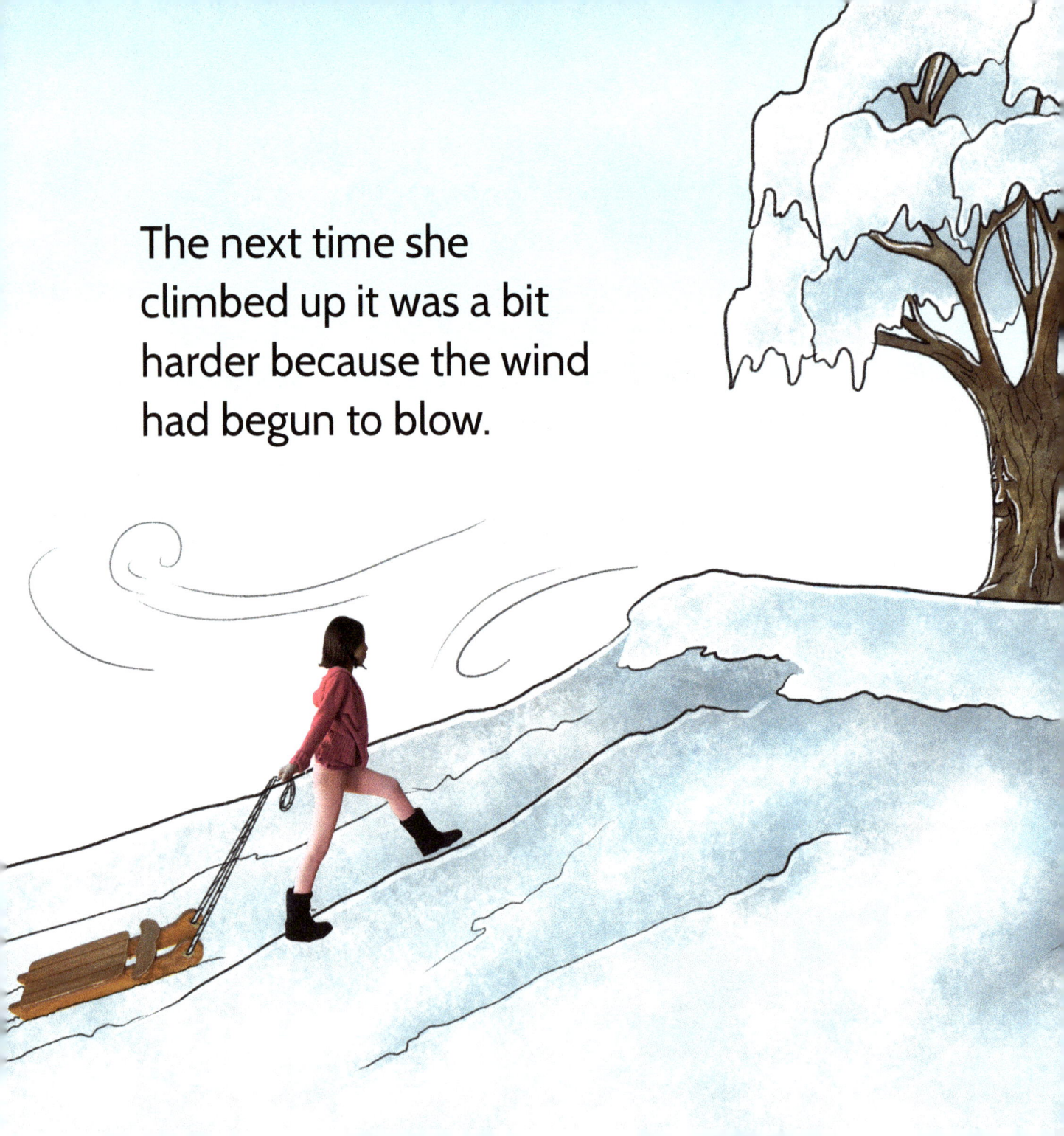

When she got to the top, the wind was very strong and she was worried. Her heart was beating hard, and she didn't know what to do.

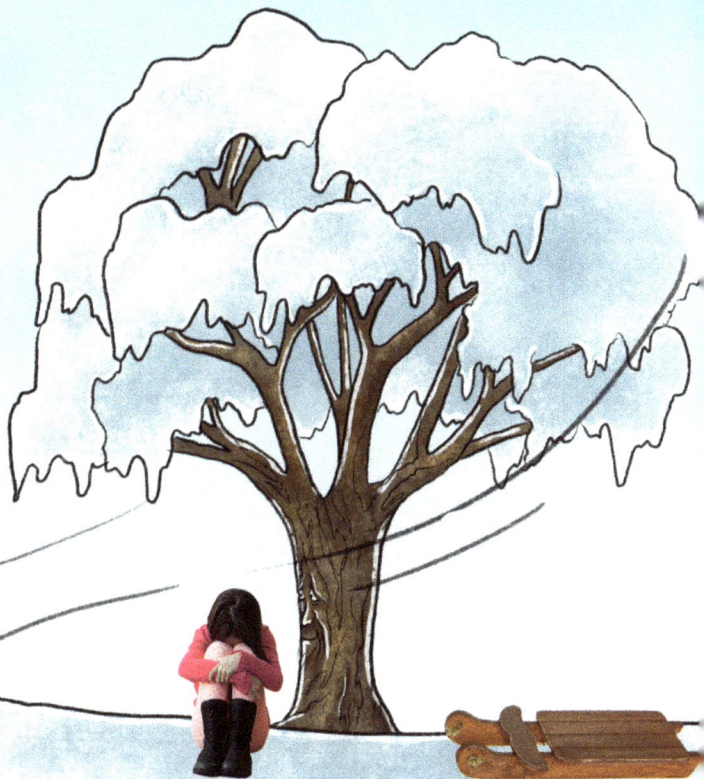

She crawled next to a nearby tree and huddled.

When the wind finally stopped, the big tree smiled at her and said, "I see you were worried in the wind. Do you want to learn how to be strong in the wind?"

Eve nodded.

"Come back tomorrow and I will show you how," said the tree.

The next morning, Eve woke up excited to go see the tree.

She stretched up and said good morning to the sun.

She put on her boots...

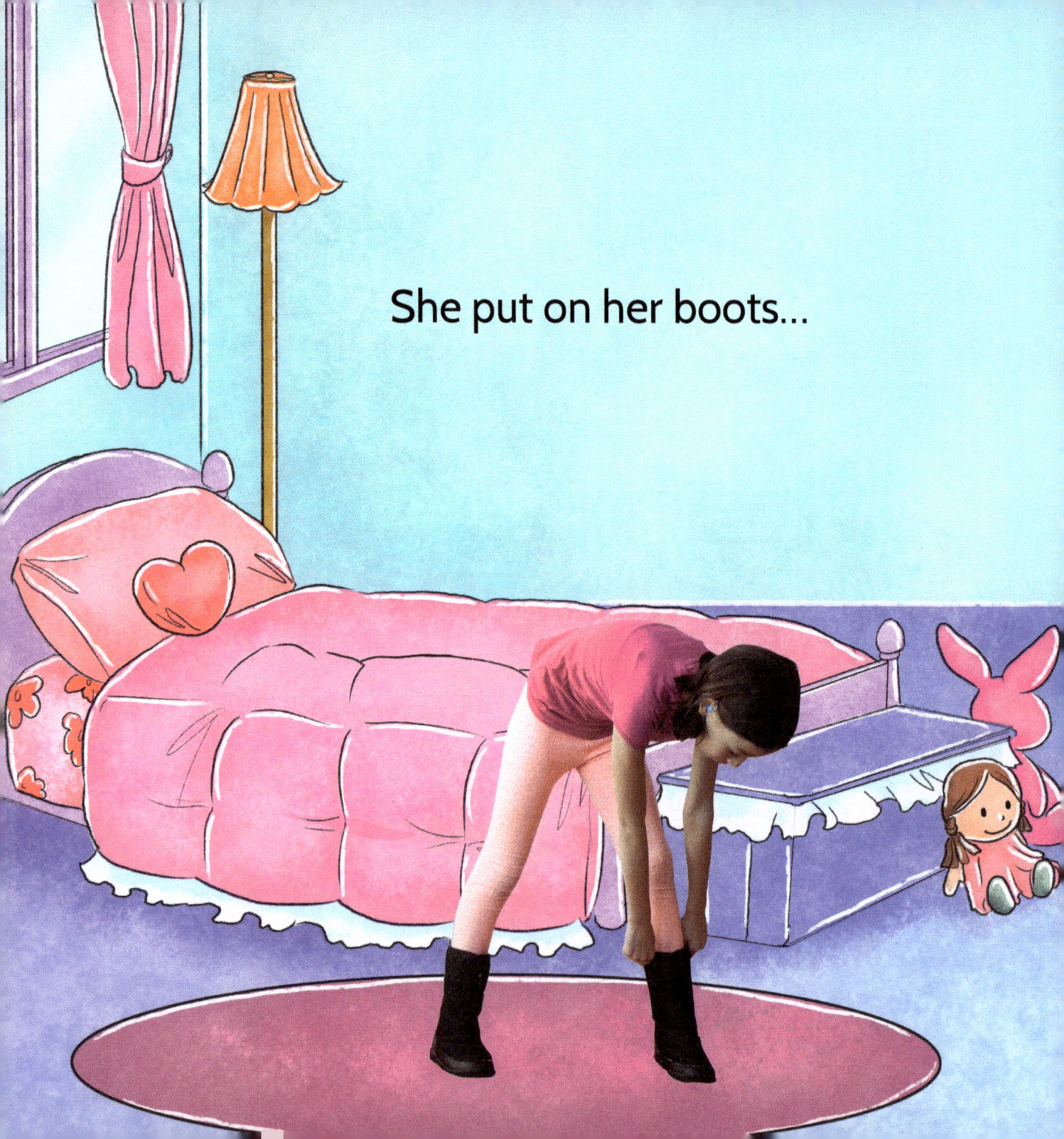

Put on her coat...

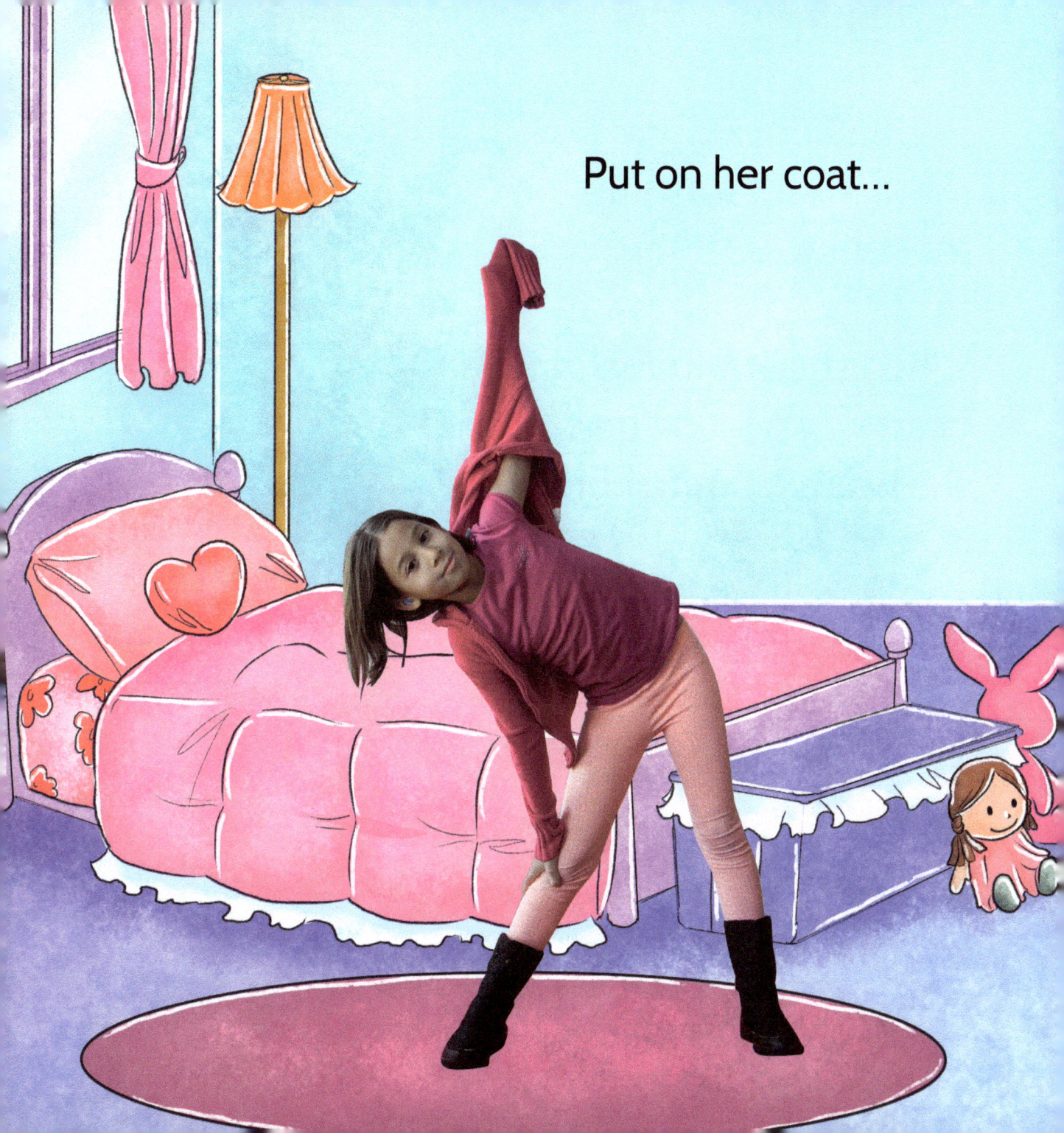

...and went up, up, up the mountain.

When she got to the top, her heart was beating quickly and she was a bit out of breath.

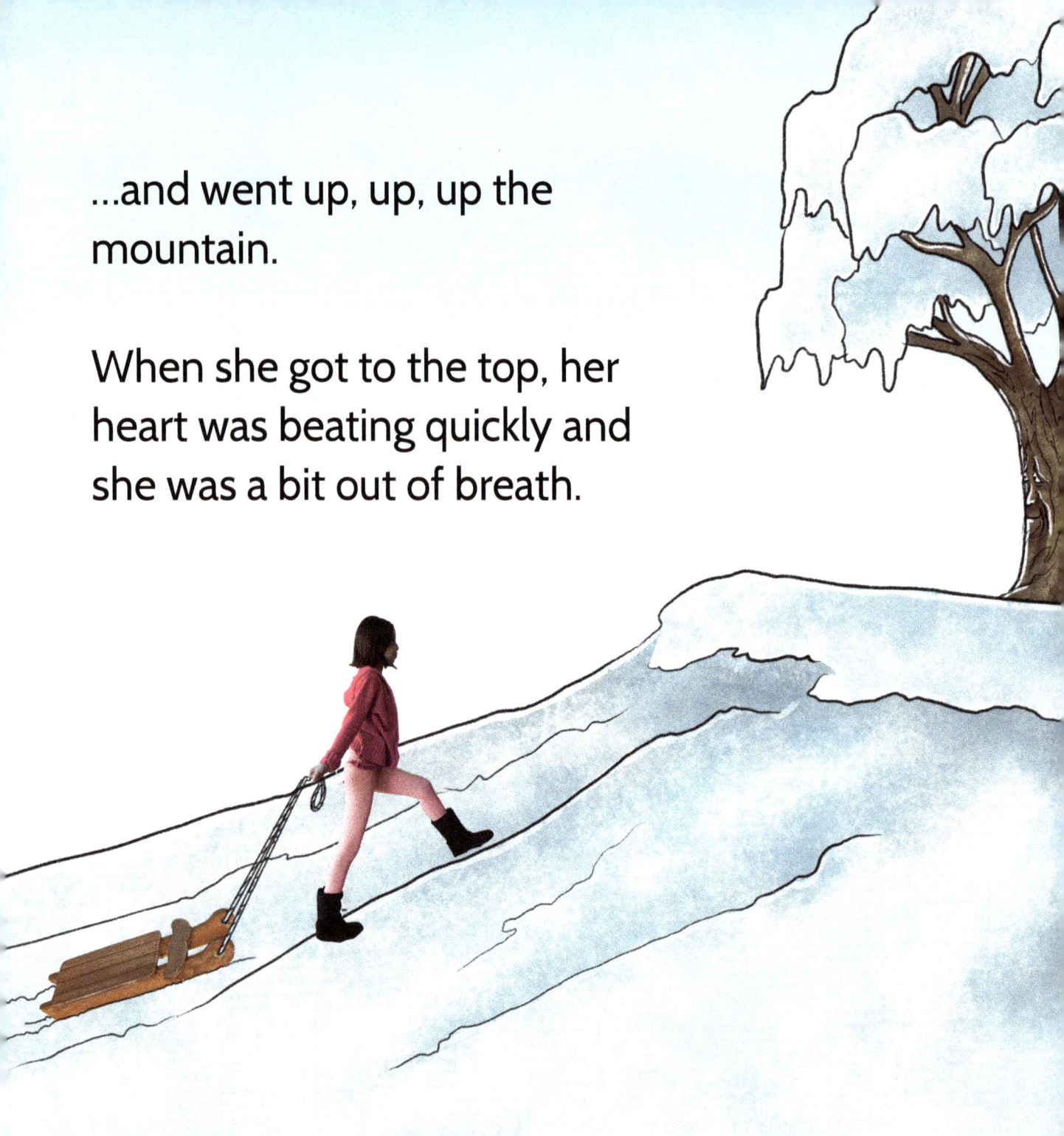

"Okay, Mr. Tree," she said, "now what should I do?"

"Sit down, and close your eyes," the tree answered. "Can you feel your heart beating? And your rapid breathing?"

"Yes," said Eve.

"Keep your eyes closed and look inside. Just keep watching and your breath and heart will eventually slow down," said the tree.

Eve did what the tree said. She watched her breath and her heart...

They eventually slowed down and she felt better.

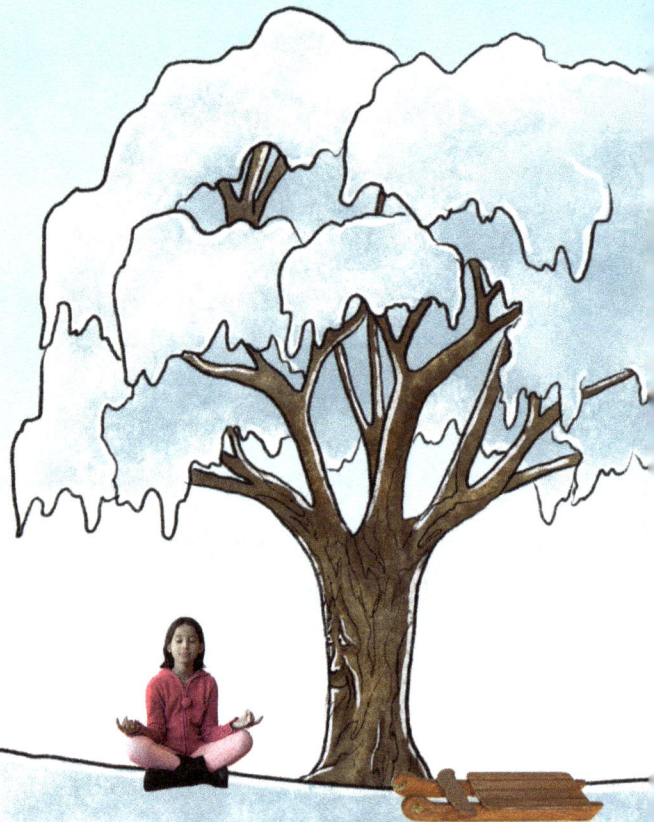

Eve was happy she had learned how to calm down.
"But can I become strong like you, Mr. Tree?" she asked.

"Of course you can," said the tree. "Just practice being like me every day."

Eve got up,
stood on one leg,
and tried to be strong
and straight
like the tree.

But she fell...

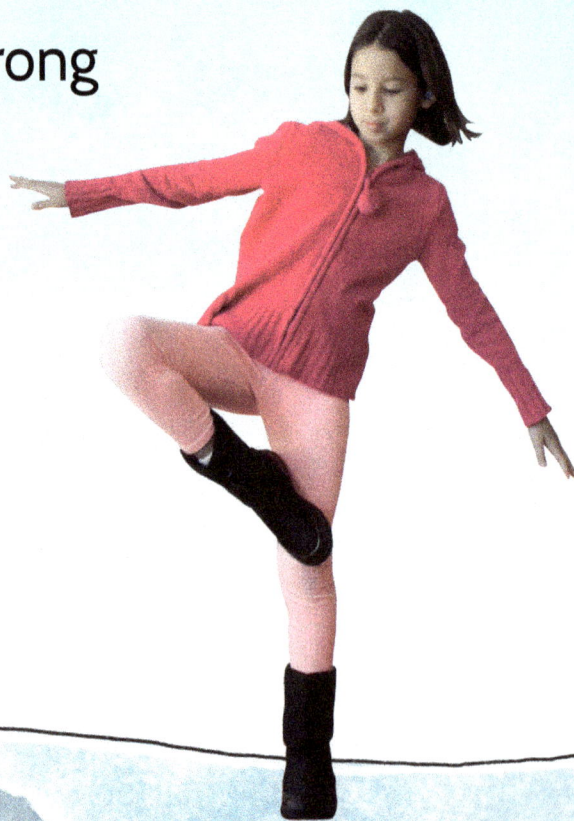

"Try again," said the tree. "Don't forget that I have roots in the ground."

"Imagine your feet are deep in the ground."

"Bravo!" said the tree. "You did it! Now open your branches."

"Remember, every tree is different from the other—with its own unique branches. You must be your *own* tree."

"And now," said the tree, "you are ready to learn how to be strong and flexible, even when the wind is blowing."

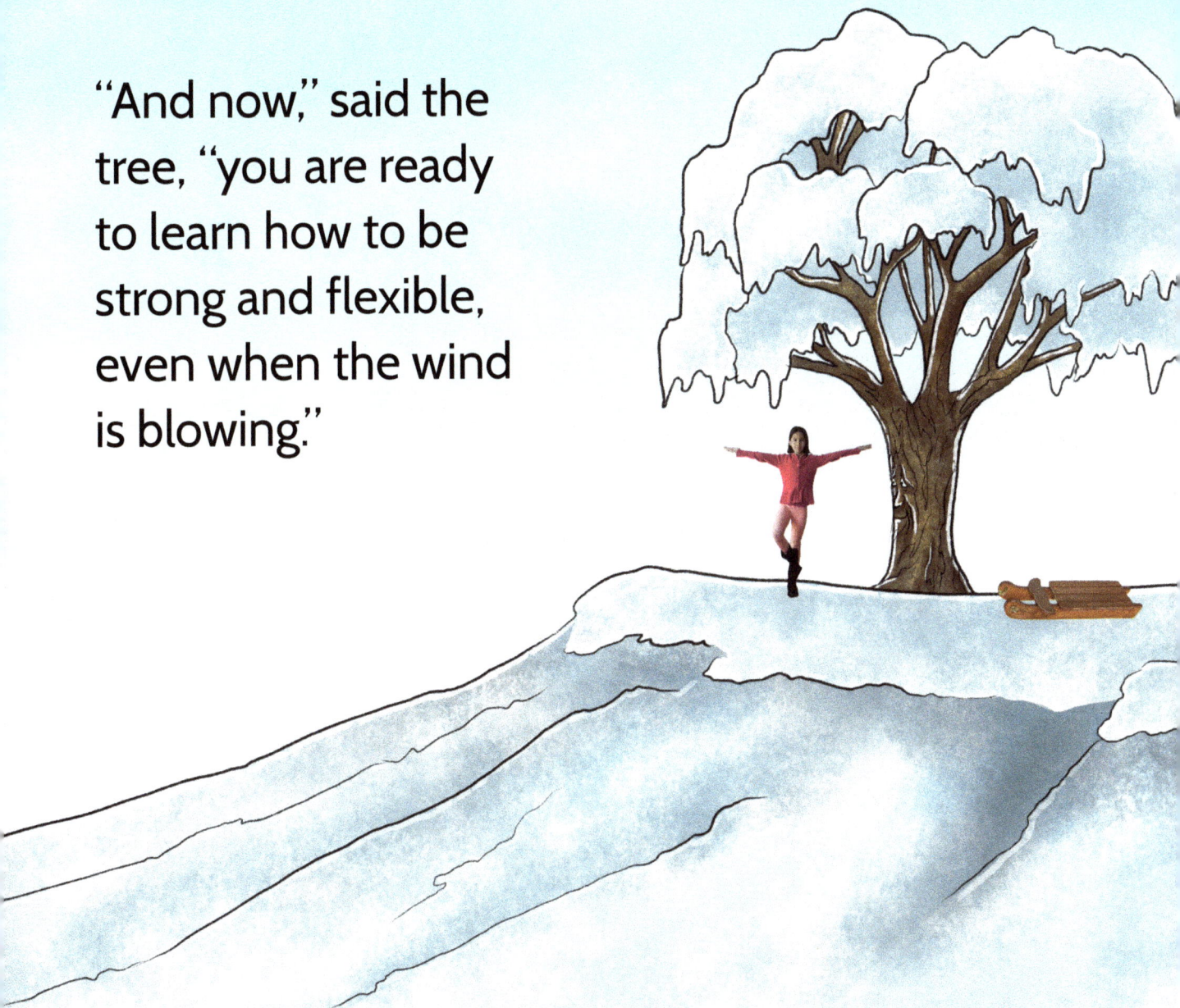

"Feel the roots in your feet, feel the wind, and bend, but don't fall!"

"Even the wind cannot topple a strong tree, as long as you are flexible with the wind."

Eve said good-bye to the tree
and walked home with a smile.

She felt stronger.

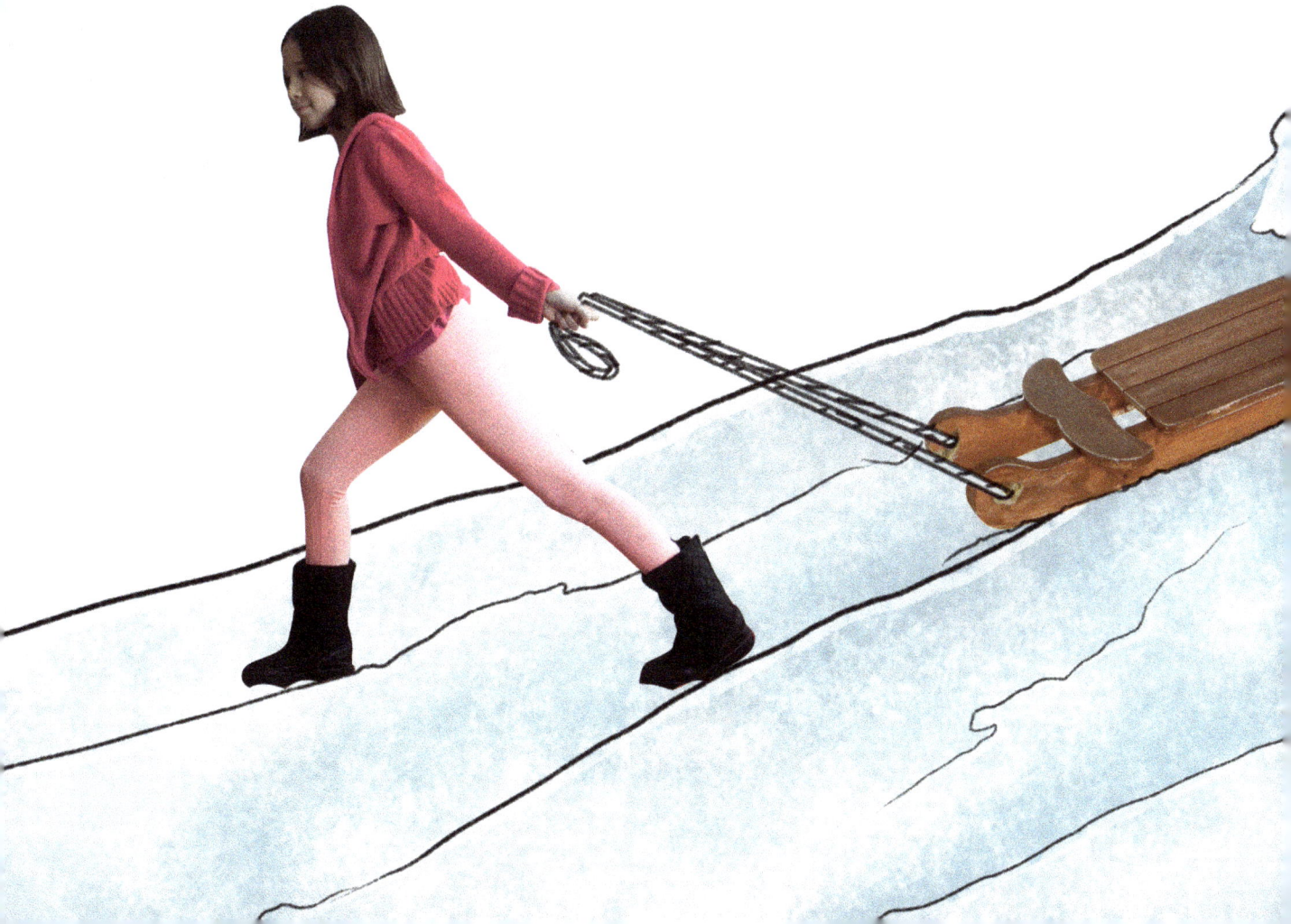

After a long day of being a tree, she lay down in her bed as happy as a baby...

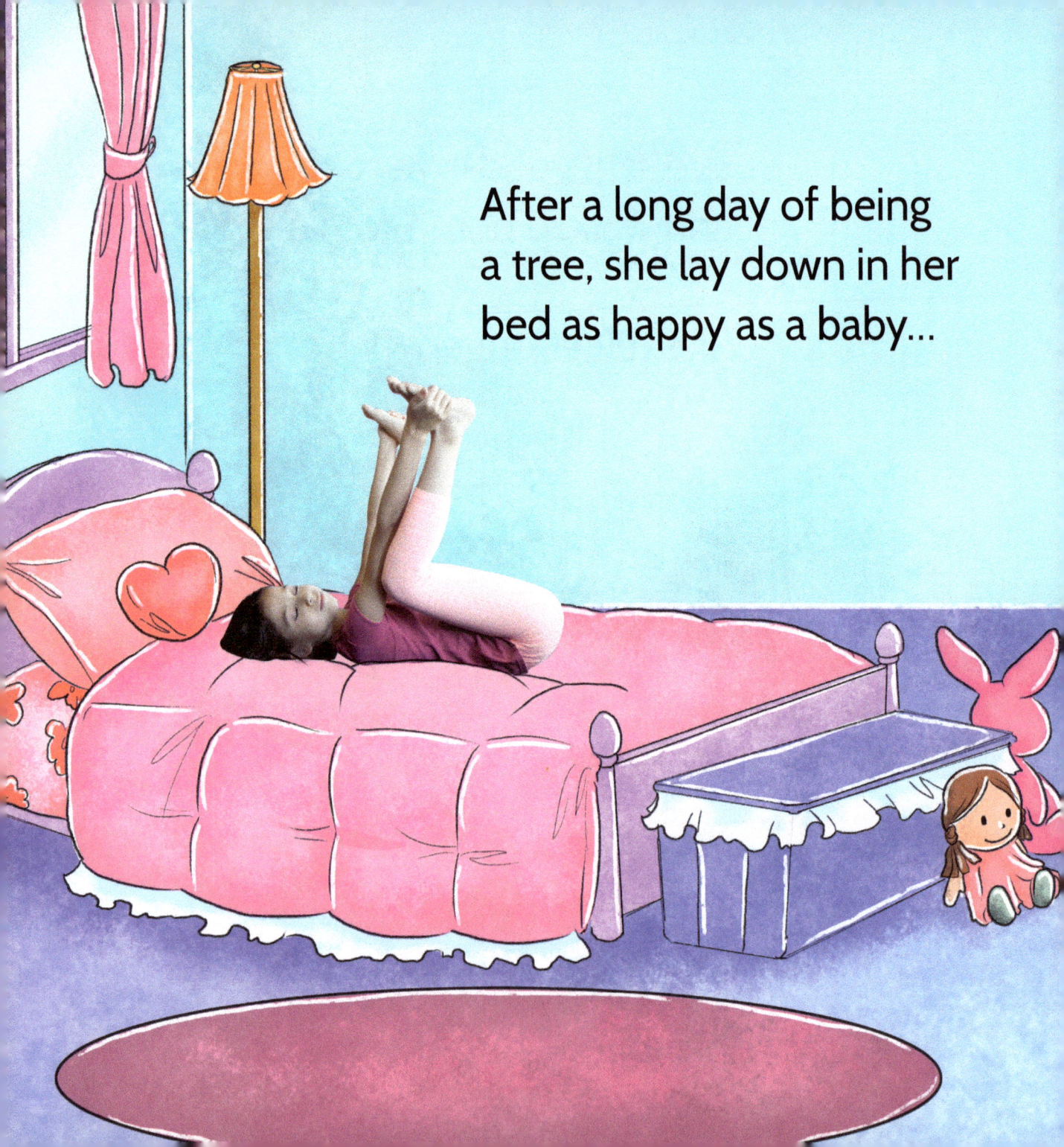

She lay on her back, closed her eyes, and took slow deep breaths.

Then she turned to her side and slid softly into her dreams.

The end

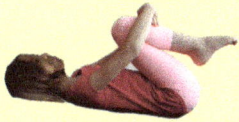

1. Knees-to-Chest Pose
Apanasana

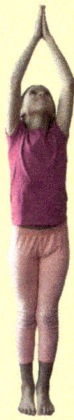

2. Extended Mountain Pose
Tadasana

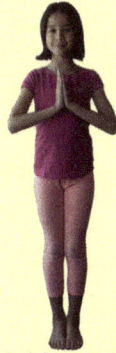

3. Mountain
Pose—Tadasana

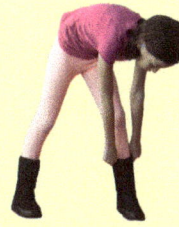

4. Intense Side Stretch Pose
Parsvottanasana

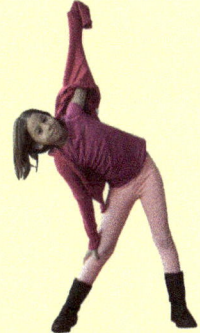

5. Triangle Pose
Utthita Trikonasana

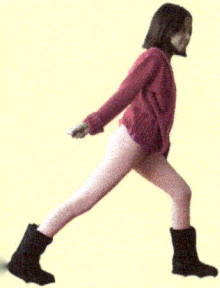

6. Lunge Pose
Anjaneyasana

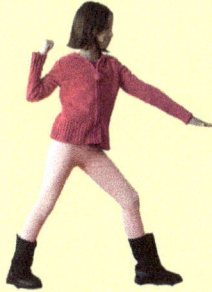

7. Warrior II Pose
Virabhadrasana II

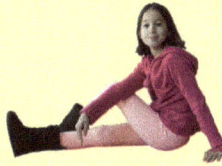

8. Half Twist Pose
Ardha Matsyendrasana

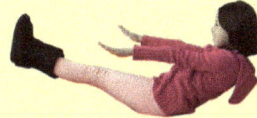

9. Boat Pose
Navasana

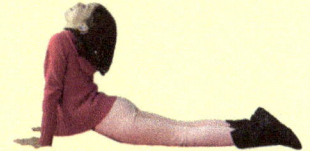

10. Upward Facing Dog Pose
Urdhva Mukha Svanasana

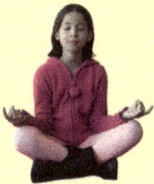

11. Easy Pose
Sukhasana

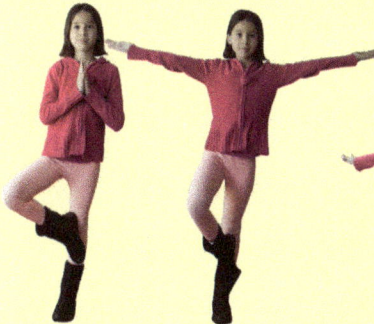

12. Tree Pose
Vrksasana

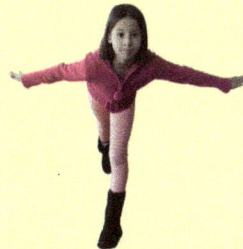

13. Toppling Tree Pose
Patanvrkshasana

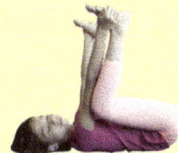

14. Happy Baby Pose
Ananda Balasana

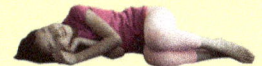

15. Fetal Pose
(after Shavasana)